This notebook belongs to:

____

Published by: Character Designs

MEDICAL HISTORY

Name:	Birth Date:
Allergies:	Blood Type:
Primary Doctor:	Contact:
Chronic Conditions:	Date:
Medications:	Note:

Date	Immunizations Illnesses, Surgeries, etc.	Notes

MEDICAL HISTORY

Name:	Birth Date:
Allergies:	Blood Type:
Primary Doctor:	Contact:
Chronic Conditions:	Date:
Medications:	Note:

Date	Immunizations Illnesses, Surgeries, etc.	Notes

MEDICAL HISTORY

Name:	Birth Date:
Allergies:	Blood Type:
Primary Doctor:	Contact:
Chronic Conditions:	Date:
Medications:	Note:

Date	Immunizations Illnesses, Surgeries, etc.	Notes

MEDICAL HISTORY

Name:	Birth Date:
Allergies:	Blood Type:
Primary Doctor:	Contact:
Chronic Conditions:	Date:
Medications:	Note:

Date	Immunizations Illnesses, Surgeries, etc.	Notes

MEDICAL HISTORY

Name:	Birth Date:
Allergies:	Blood Type:
Primary Doctor:	Contact:
Chronic Conditions:	Date:
Medications:	Note:

Date	Immunizations Illnesses, Surgeries, etc.	Notes

MEDICAL HISTORY

Name:	Birth Date:
Allergies:	Blood Type:
Primary Doctor:	Contact:
Chronic Conditions:	Date:
Medications:	Note:

Date	Immunizations Illnesses, Surgeries, etc.	Notes

MEDICAL HISTORY

Name:	Birth Date:
Allergies:	Blood Type:
Primary Doctor:	Contact:
Chronic Conditions:	Date:
Medications:	Note:

Date	Immunizations Illnesses, Surgeries, etc.	Notes

MEDICAL HISTORY

Name:	Birth Date:
Allergies:	Blood Type:
Primary Doctor:	Contact:
Chronic Conditions:	Date:
Medications:	Note:

Date	Immunizations Illnesses, Surgeries, etc.	Notes

MEDICAL HISTORY

Name:	Birth Date:
Allergies:	Blood Type:
Primary Doctor:	Contact:
Chronic Conditions:	Date:
Medications:	Note:

Date	Immunizations Illnesses, Surgeries, etc.	Notes

MEDICAL HISTORY

Name:	Birth Date:
Allergies:	Blood Type:
Primary Doctor:	Contact:
Chronic Conditions:	Date:
Medications:	Note:

Date	Immunizations Illnesses, Surgeries, etc.	Notes

MEDICAL HISTORY

Name:	Birth Date:
Allergies:	Blood Type:
Primary Doctor:	Contact:
Chronic Conditions:	Date:
Medications:	Note:

Date	Immunizations Illnesses, Surgeries, etc.	Notes

MEDICAL HISTORY

Name:	Birth Date:
Allergies:	Blood Type:
Primary Doctor:	Contact:
Chronic Conditions:	Date:
Medications:	Note:

Date	Immunizations Illnesses, Surgeries, etc.	Notes

MEDICAL HISTORY

Name:	Birth Date:
Allergies:	Blood Type:
Primary Doctor:	Contact:
Chronic Conditions:	Date:
Medications:	Note:

Date	Immunizations Illnesses, Surgeries, etc.	Notes

MEDICAL HISTORY

Name:	Birth Date:
Allergies:	Blood Type:
Primary Doctor:	Contact:
Chronic Conditions:	Date:
Medications:	Note:

Date	Immunizations Illnesses, Surgeries, etc.	Notes

MEDICAL HISTORY

Name:	Birth Date:
Allergies:	Blood Type:
Primary Doctor:	Contact:
Chronic Conditions:	Date:
Medications:	Note:

Date	Immunizations Illnesses, Surgeries, etc.	Notes

MEDICAL HISTORY

Name:	Birth Date:
Allergies:	Blood Type:
Primary Doctor:	Contact:
Chronic Conditions:	Date:
Medications:	Note:

Date	Immunizations Illnesses, Surgeries, etc.	Notes

MEDICAL HISTORY

Name:	Birth Date:
Allergies:	Blood Type:
Primary Doctor:	Contact:
Chronic Conditions:	Date:
Medications:	Note:

Date	Immunizations Illnesses, Surgeries, etc.	Notes

MEDICAL HISTORY

Name:	Birth Date:
Allergies:	Blood Type:
Primary Doctor:	Contact:
Chronic Conditions:	Date:
Medications:	Note:

Date	Immunizations Illnesses, Surgeries, etc.	Notes

MEDICAL HISTORY

Name:	Birth Date:
Allergies:	Blood Type:
Primary Doctor:	Contact:
Chronic Conditions:	Date:
Medications:	Note:

Date	Immunizations Illnesses, Surgeries, etc.	Notes

MEDICAL HISTORY

Name:	Birth Date:
Allergies:	Blood Type:
Primary Doctor:	Contact:
Chronic Conditions:	Date:
Medications:	Note:

Date	Immunizations Illnesses, Surgeries, etc.	Notes

MEDICAL HISTORY

Name:	Birth Date:
Allergies:	Blood Type:
Primary Doctor:	Contact:
Chronic Conditions:	Date:
Medications:	Note:

Date	Immunizations Illnesses, Surgeries, etc.	Notes

MEDICAL HISTORY

Name:	Birth Date:
Allergies:	Blood Type:
Primary Doctor:	Contact:
Chronic Conditions:	Date:
Medications:	Note:

Date	Immunizations Illnesses, Surgeries, etc.	Notes

MEDICAL HISTORY

Name:	Birth Date:
Allergies:	Blood Type:
Primary Doctor:	Contact:
Chronic Conditions:	Date:
Medications:	Note:

Date	Immunizations Illnesses, Surgeries, etc.	Notes

MEDICAL HISTORY

Name:	Birth Date:
Allergies:	Blood Type:
Primary Doctor:	Contact:
Chronic Conditions:	Date:
Medications:	Note:

Date	Immunizations Illnesses, Surgeries, etc.	Notes

MEDICAL HISTORY

Name:	Birth Date:
Allergies:	Blood Type:
Primary Doctor:	Contact:
Chronic Conditions:	Date:
Medications:	Note:

Date	Immunizations Illnesses, Surgeries, etc.	Notes

MEDICAL HISTORY

Name:		Birth Date:
Allergies:		Blood Type:
Primary Doctor:		Contact:
Chronic Conditions:		Date:
Medications:		Note:

Date	Immunizations Illnesses, Surgeries, etc.	Notes

MEDICAL HISTORY

Name:	Birth Date:
Allergies:	Blood Type:
Primary Doctor:	Contact:
Chronic Conditions:	Date:
Medications:	Note:

Date	Immunizations Illnesses, Surgeries, etc.	Notes

MEDICAL HISTORY

Name:	Birth Date:
Allergies:	Blood Type:
Primary Doctor:	Contact:
Chronic Conditions:	Date:
Medications:	Note:

Date	Immunizations Illnesses, Surgeries, etc.	Notes

MEDICAL HISTORY

Name:	Birth Date:
Allergies:	Blood Type:
Primary Doctor:	Contact:
Chronic Conditions:	Date:
Medications:	Note:

Date	Immunizations Illnesses, Surgeries, etc.	Notes

MEDICAL HISTORY

Name:	Birth Date:
Allergies:	Blood Type:
Primary Doctor:	Contact:
Chronic Conditions:	Date:
Medications:	Note:

Date	Immunizations Illnesses, Surgeries, etc.	Notes

MEDICAL HISTORY

Name:	Birth Date:
Allergies:	Blood Type:
Primary Doctor:	Contact:
Chronic Conditions:	Date:
Medications:	Note:

Date	Immunizations Illnesses, Surgeries, etc.	Notes

MEDICAL HISTORY

Name:	Birth Date:
Allergies:	Blood Type:
Primary Doctor:	Contact:
Chronic Conditions:	Date:
Medications:	Note:

Date	Immunizations Illnesses, Surgeries, etc.	Notes

MEDICAL HISTORY

Name:	Birth Date:
Allergies:	Blood Type:
Primary Doctor:	Contact:
Chronic Conditions:	Date:
Medications:	Note:

Date	Immunizations Illnesses, Surgeries, etc.	Notes

MEDICAL HISTORY

Name:	Birth Date:
Allergies:	Blood Type:
Primary Doctor:	Contact:
Chronic Conditions:	Date:
Medications:	Note:

Date	Immunizations Illnesses, Surgeries, etc.	Notes

MEDICAL HISTORY

Name:	Birth Date:
Allergies:	Blood Type:
Primary Doctor:	Contact:
Chronic Conditions:	Date:
Medications:	Note:

Date	Immunizations Illnesses, Surgeries, etc.	Notes

MEDICAL HISTORY

Name:	Birth Date:
Allergies:	Blood Type:
Primary Doctor:	Contact:
Chronic Conditions:	Date:
Medications:	Note:

Date	Immunizations Illnesses, Surgeries, etc.	Notes

MEDICAL HISTORY

Name:	Birth Date:
Allergies:	Blood Type:
Primary Doctor:	Contact:
Chronic Conditions:	Date:
Medications:	Note:

Date	Immunizations Illnesses, Surgeries, etc.	Notes

MEDICAL HISTORY

Name:	Birth Date:
Allergies:	Blood Type:
Primary Doctor:	Contact:
Chronic Conditions:	Date:
Medications:	Note:

Date	Immunizations Illnesses, Surgeries, etc.	Notes

MEDICAL HISTORY

Name:	Birth Date:
Allergies:	Blood Type:
Primary Doctor:	Contact:
Chronic Conditions:	Date:
Medications:	Note:

Date	Immunizations Illnesses, Surgeries, etc.	Notes

MEDICAL HISTORY

Name:	Birth Date:
Allergies:	Blood Type:
Primary Doctor:	Contact:
Chronic Conditions:	Date:
Medications:	Note:

Date	Immunizations Illnesses, Surgeries, etc.	Notes

MEDICAL HISTORY

Name:	Birth Date:
Allergies:	Blood Type:
Primary Doctor:	Contact:
Chronic Conditions:	Date:
Medications:	Note:

Date	Immunizations Illnesses, Surgeries, etc.	Notes

MEDICAL HISTORY

Name:	Birth Date:
Allergies:	Blood Type:
Primary Doctor:	Contact:
Chronic Conditions:	Date:
Medications:	Note:

Date	Immunizations Illnesses, Surgeries, etc.	Notes

MEDICAL HISTORY

Name:	Birth Date:
Allergies:	Blood Type:
Primary Doctor:	Contact:
Chronic Conditions:	Date:
Medications:	Note:

Date	Immunizations Illnesses, Surgeries, etc.	Notes

MEDICAL HISTORY

Name:	Birth Date:
Allergies:	Blood Type:
Primary Doctor:	Contact:
Chronic Conditions:	Date:
Medications:	Note:

Date	Immunizations Illnesses, Surgeries, etc.	Notes

MEDICAL HISTORY

Name:	Birth Date:
Allergies:	Blood Type:
Primary Doctor:	Contact:
Chronic Conditions:	Date:
Medications:	Note:

Date	Immunizations Illnesses, Surgeries, etc.	Notes

MEDICAL HISTORY

Name:	Birth Date:
Allergies:	Blood Type:
Primary Doctor:	Contact:
Chronic Conditions:	Date:
Medications:	Note:

Date	Immunizations Illnesses, Surgeries, etc.	Notes

MEDICAL HISTORY

Name:	Birth Date:
Allergies:	Blood Type:
Primary Doctor:	Contact:
Chronic Conditions:	Date:
Medications:	Note:

Date	Immunizations Illnesses, Surgeries, etc.	Notes

MEDICAL HISTORY

Name:	Birth Date:
Allergies:	Blood Type:
Primary Doctor:	Contact:
Chronic Conditions:	Date:
Medications:	Note:

Date	Immunizations Illnesses, Surgeries, etc.	Notes

MEDICAL HISTORY

Name:	Birth Date:
Allergies:	Blood Type:
Primary Doctor:	Contact:
Chronic Conditions:	Date:
Medications:	Note:

Date	Immunizations Illnesses, Surgeries, etc.	Notes

MEDICAL HISTORY

Name:	Birth Date:
Allergies:	Blood Type:
Primary Doctor:	Contact:
Chronic Conditions:	Date:
Medications:	Note:

Date	Immunizations Illnesses, Surgeries, etc.	Notes

MEDICAL HISTORY

Name:	Birth Date:
Allergies:	Blood Type:
Primary Doctor:	Contact:
Chronic Conditions:	Date:
Medications:	Note:

Date	Immunizations Illnesses, Surgeries, etc.	Notes

MEDICAL HISTORY

Name:	Birth Date:
Allergies:	Blood Type:
Primary Doctor:	Contact:
Chronic Conditions:	Date:
Medications:	Note:

Date	Immunizations Illnesses, Surgeries, etc.	Notes

MEDICAL HISTORY

Name:	Birth Date:
Allergies:	Blood Type:
Primary Doctor:	Contact:
Chronic Conditions:	Date:
Medications:	Note:

Date	Immunizations Illnesses, Surgeries, etc.	Notes

MEDICAL HISTORY

Name:	Birth Date:
Allergies:	Blood Type:
Primary Doctor:	Contact:
Chronic Conditions:	Date:
Medications:	Note:

Date	Immunizations Illnesses, Surgeries, etc.	Notes

MEDICAL HISTORY

Name:	Birth Date:
Allergies:	Blood Type:
Primary Doctor:	Contact:
Chronic Conditions:	Date:
Medications:	Note:

Date	Immunizations Illnesses, Surgeries, etc.	Notes

MEDICAL HISTORY

Name:	Birth Date:
Allergies:	Blood Type:
Primary Doctor:	Contact:
Chronic Conditions:	Date:
Medications:	Note:

Date	Immunizations Illnesses, Surgeries, etc.	Notes

MEDICAL HISTORY

Name:	Birth Date:
Allergies:	Blood Type:
Primary Doctor:	Contact:
Chronic Conditions:	Date:
Medications:	Note:

Date	Immunizations Illnesses, Surgeries, etc.	Notes

MEDICAL HISTORY

Name:	Birth Date:
Allergies:	Blood Type:
Primary Doctor:	Contact:
Chronic Conditions:	Date:
Medications:	Note:

Date	Immunizations Illnesses, Surgeries, etc.	Notes

MEDICAL HISTORY

Name:	Birth Date:
Allergies:	Blood Type:
Primary Doctor:	Contact:
Chronic Conditions:	Date:
Medications:	Note:

Date	Immunizations Illnesses, Surgeries, etc.	Notes

MEDICAL HISTORY

<table>
<tr><td>Name:</td><td>Birth Date:</td></tr>
<tr><td>Allergies:</td><td>Blood Type:</td></tr>
<tr><td>Primary Doctor:</td><td>Contact:</td></tr>
<tr><td>Chronic Conditions:</td><td>Date:</td></tr>
<tr><td>Medications:</td><td>Note:</td></tr>
</table>

Date	Immunizations Illnesses, Surgeries, etc.	Notes

MEDICAL HISTORY

Name:	Birth Date:
Allergies:	Blood Type:
Primary Doctor:	Contact:
Chronic Conditions:	Date:
Medications:	Note:

Date	Immunizations Illnesses, Surgeries, etc.	Notes

MEDICAL HISTORY

Name:	Birth Date:
Allergies:	Blood Type:
Primary Doctor:	Contact:
Chronic Conditions:	Date:
Medications:	Note:

Date	Immunizations Illnesses, Surgeries, etc.	Notes

MEDICAL HISTORY

Name:	Birth Date:
Allergies:	Blood Type:
Primary Doctor:	Contact:
Chronic Conditions:	Date:
Medications:	Note:

Date	Immunizations Illnesses, Surgeries, etc.	Notes

MEDICAL HISTORY

Name:	Birth Date:
Allergies:	Blood Type:
Primary Doctor:	Contact:
Chronic Conditions:	Date:
Medications:	Note:

Date	Immunizations Illnesses, Surgeries, etc.	Notes

MEDICAL HISTORY

Name:	Birth Date:
Allergies:	Blood Type:
Primary Doctor:	Contact:
Chronic Conditions:	Date:
Medications:	Note:

Date	Immunizations Illnesses, Surgeries, etc.	Notes

MEDICAL HISTORY

Name:	Birth Date:
Allergies:	Blood Type:
Primary Doctor:	Contact:
Chronic Conditions:	Date:
Medications:	Note:

Date	Immunizations Illnesses, Surgeries, etc.	Notes

MEDICAL HISTORY

Name:	Birth Date:
Allergies:	Blood Type:
Primary Doctor:	Contact:
Chronic Conditions:	Date:
Medications:	Note:

Date	Immunizations Illnesses, Surgeries, etc.	Notes

MEDICAL HISTORY

Name:	Birth Date:
Allergies:	Blood Type:
Primary Doctor:	Contact:
Chronic Conditions:	Date:
Medications:	Note:

Date	Immunizations Illnesses, Surgeries, etc.	Notes

MEDICAL HISTORY

Name:	Birth Date:
Allergies:	Blood Type:
Primary Doctor:	Contact:
Chronic Conditions:	Date:
Medications:	Note:

Date	Immunizations Illnesses, Surgeries, etc.	Notes

MEDICAL HISTORY

Name:	Birth Date:
Allergies:	Blood Type:
Primary Doctor:	Contact:
Chronic Conditions:	Date:
Medications:	Note:

Date	Immunizations Illnesses, Surgeries, etc.	Notes

MEDICAL HISTORY

Name:	Birth Date:
Allergies:	Blood Type:
Primary Doctor:	Contact:
Chronic Conditions:	Date:
Medications:	Note:

Date	Immunizations Illnesses, Surgeries, etc.	Notes

MEDICAL HISTORY

Name:	Birth Date:
Allergies:	Blood Type:
Primary Doctor:	Contact:
Chronic Conditions:	Date:
Medications:	Note:

Date	Immunizations Illnesses, Surgeries, etc.	Notes

MEDICAL HISTORY

Name:		Birth Date:
Allergies:		Blood Type:
Primary Doctor:		Contact:
Chronic Conditions:		Date:
Medications:		Note:

Date	Immunizations Illnesses, Surgeries, etc.	Notes

MEDICAL HISTORY

Name:	Birth Date:
Allergies:	Blood Type:
Primary Doctor:	Contact:
Chronic Conditions:	Date:
Medications:	Note:

Date	Immunizations Illnesses, Surgeries, etc.	Notes

MEDICAL HISTORY

Name:	Birth Date:
Allergies:	Blood Type:
Primary Doctor:	Contact:
Chronic Conditions:	Date:
Medications:	Note:

Date	Immunizations Illnesses, Surgeries, etc.	Notes

MEDICAL HISTORY

Name:	Birth Date:
Allergies:	Blood Type:
Primary Doctor:	Contact:
Chronic Conditions:	Date:
Medications:	Note:

Date	Immunizations Illnesses, Surgeries, etc.	Notes

MEDICAL HISTORY

Name:	Birth Date:
Allergies:	Blood Type:
Primary Doctor:	Contact:
Chronic Conditions:	Date:
Medications:	Note:

Date	Immunizations Illnesses, Surgeries, etc.	Notes

MEDICAL HISTORY

Name:	Birth Date:
Allergies:	Blood Type:
Primary Doctor:	Contact:
Chronic Conditions:	Date:
Medications:	Note:

Date	Immunizations Illnesses, Surgeries, etc.	Notes

MEDICAL HISTORY

Name:	Birth Date:
Allergies:	Blood Type:
Primary Doctor:	Contact:
Chronic Conditions:	Date:
Medications:	Note:

Date	Immunizations Illnesses, Surgeries, etc.	Notes

MEDICAL HISTORY

Name:	Birth Date:
Allergies:	Blood Type:
Primary Doctor:	Contact:
Chronic Conditions:	Date:
Medications:	Note:

Date	Immunizations Illnesses, Surgeries, etc.	Notes

Takeaway notes:

Year of use: